D1367298

Weekly Reader Books presents

What to do when your mom or dad says . . . "BE PREPARED!"

By

JOY WILT BERRY

Living Skills Press
Fallbrook, California

Weekly Reader Books edition published by
arrangement with Living Skills Press.

Dear Parents,

"BE PREPARED!" Have you ever made this urgent request and had your child respond with a yawn and a glance that said: "How come you're so uptight?"

It's obvious that you know something that your child doesn't know. You, through experience, have learned that the world "as it really is" isn't always as snug and safe as the world your child has experienced during the early years of life. You know that there are things out there that will "get ya if ya don't watch out!"

But, how do you tell your child about these things? Up to now you've probably done everything you could to protect your child. You've bent over backwards to keep your child safe and as free as possible from any amount of pain. How can you possibly tell your child about kidnapping, tornadoes, and accidents without scaring him or her to death or causing nightmares? No one wants to scare a child unduly, but the fact is, to deal with real life, your child needs to know about it.

The bad news is there are things in the world that can hurt us. The good news is "most likely, we can handle them." The trick is to learn how.

Handling difficult situations begins with a respect for them. This respect may involve a healthy amount of fear. Fear at its best causes a person to be careful in situations that demand caution. Thus your child should be encouraged to listen and respond to his or her fears. Oftentimes a child has already accumulated a set of "healthy fears"; other times, parents have to assist a child in acquiring them. A lot of a child's unnecessary fear comes from "not knowing." All too often a child fears things he or she does not know about. The child fills in the empty blanks with irrational answers and ...

these answers lead to illogical behavior. When this happens, the child needs to be educated so that any unnecessary fear can be dissipated. The only fear that needs to be preserved and respected is well-founded fear. You will need to exercise great care in helping your child sort through these fears.

Once a child is respectful of difficult situations, he or she must learn the specifics of dealing with them. Here's where this book comes in. It can be most helpful in explaining exactly what needs to be done in difficult situations. More importantly it will tell children why something must be done.

If you will use the book systematically (as part of a continuing program or as a resource to be used whenever the need for it arises), you and your child will experience some very positive results.

With your help your child will "BE PREPARED!"

Sincerely,

Joy Wilt Berry

Has your mother or father ever told you to ...

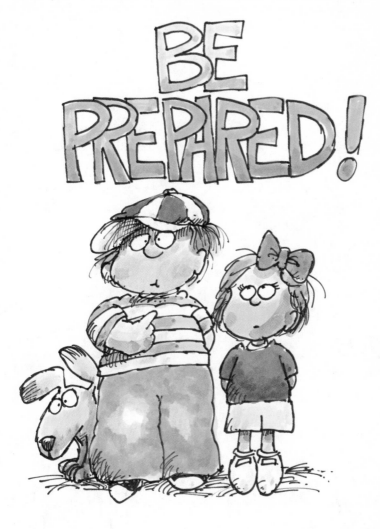

BE PREPARED!

Whenever you are told to be prepared, do you ever wonder ...

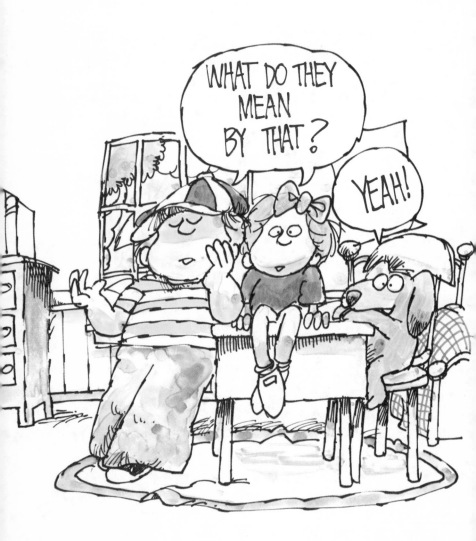

If any of this sounds familiar to you, you're going to *love* this book!

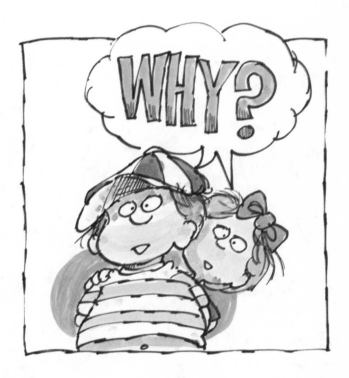

Because it will tell you exactly what it means and what to do to be prepared. If you will follow the instructions outlined in this book, you will be prepared to face the emergencies that may happen.

Sometime during your childhood you may be involved in an emergency. An emergency is something that happens suddenly and needs attention right away.

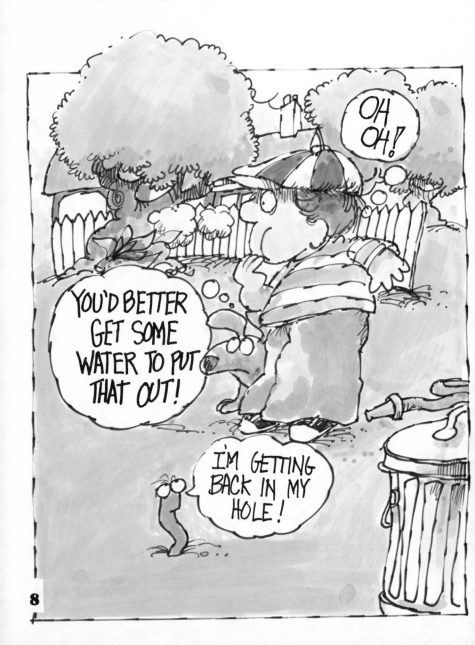

You will be able to handle some emergencies on your own, but you might need help handling others.

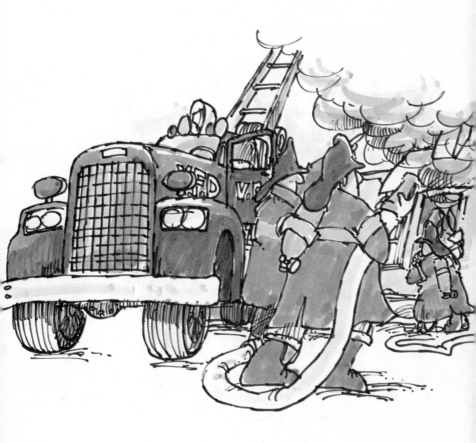

The purpose of this book is to get you ready to handle emergencies **before** they happen.

THINGS YOU NEED TO KNOW ABOUT YOURSELF

Sometime you may find yourself in an emergency in which you need someone else to help you. You may need to give that person some information about yourself.

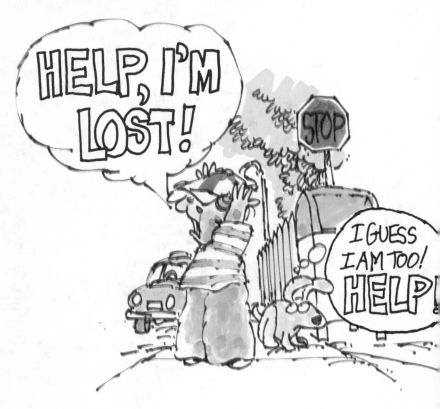

You will probably be asked for:

— your FULL NAME (your first, middle, and last name).

— your ADDRESS (your house number, the name of the street you live on, and city and state you live in).

— your TELEPHONE NUMBER (the area code and telephone number).

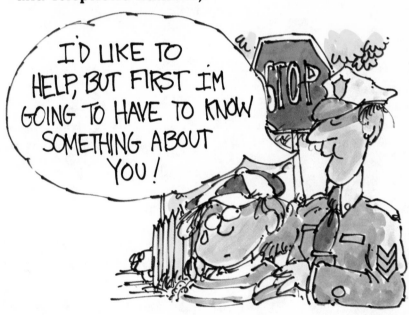

I'D LIKE TO HELP, BUT FIRST I'M GOING TO HAVE TO KNOW SOMETHING ABOUT YOU!

So that you will be able to give this information whenever it is necessary, write it down here, and then memorize it.

Your Name:

_____

First   Middle   Last

Your Address:

_____

Your house number   Name of your street   Name of your city or
                                                     town and state

_____

Your zip code   Your telephone number
                         Area code   Telephone number

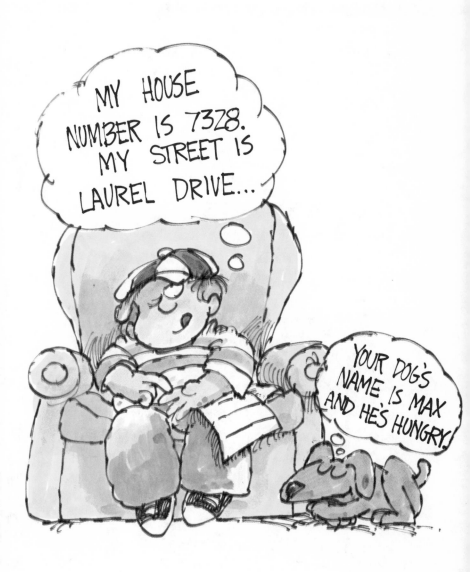

THINGS YOU NEED TO KNOW ABOUT PARENTS (OR GUARDIANS)

You may need to give the person who is helping you information about your parents.

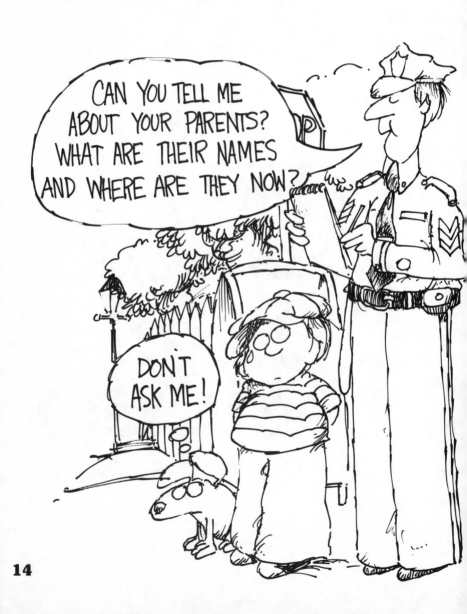

You will probably be asked for:

— your parents' full names (including their first, middle, and last name).

— your parents' address (the house number, the name of the street they live on, and the city and state they live in).

— the names and addresses of the places where your parents work.

— their telephone numbers (both at home and at work).

So you will be able to give this information whenever necessary, write it down here and memorize it.

INFORMATION ABOUT YOUR FATHER OR MALE GUARDIAN

His Name:

_____

First   Middle   Last

His Address:

_____

His house number   Name of his street   Name of his city and state

Where He Works:

_____

Name of the place   Address of the place   Name of the city
where he works   where he works   where he works

His home telephone number: His work telephone number:

_____

INFORMATION ABOUT YOUR MOTHER OR FEMALE GUARDIAN

Her Name:

_____

First   Middle   Last

Her Address:

_____

Her house number   Name of her street   Name of her city and state

Where She Works:

_____

Name of the place   Address of the place   Name of the city
where she works   where she works   where she works

Her home telephone number: Her work telephone number:

_____

THINGS YOUR PARENTS OR GUARDIANS NEED TO KNOW WHENEVER YOU ARE AWAY FROM THEM

You may encounter an emergency when you are away from your parents or guardians.

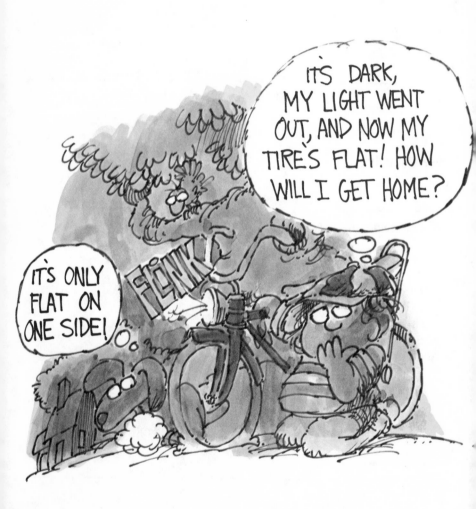

If your parents or guardians are to help you, they will need to know where you are.

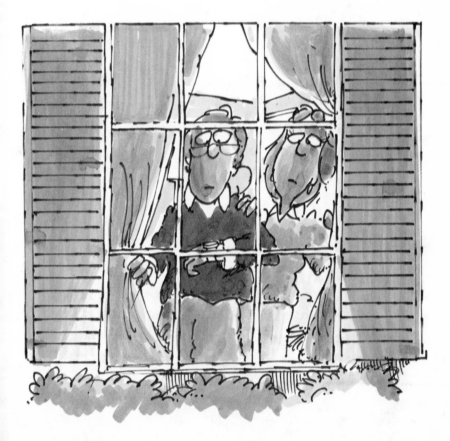

Before you leave your parents or guardians, be sure that they know:

— where you will be (the name, address, and telephone number of the place),

— what you will be doing,

— how you will get there (Who will take you? Who will bring you home? Will you be walking or riding your bike? Tell them the route you will take if you plan to walk or ride your bike),

— when you plan to return.

It's a good idea to have an emergency sheet like this posted by your list of emergency telephone numbers so that you will be sure to give all of the correct information.

When you are away from your parents or guardians, it's very important that you make sure they know exactly where you are and what you are doing at all times.

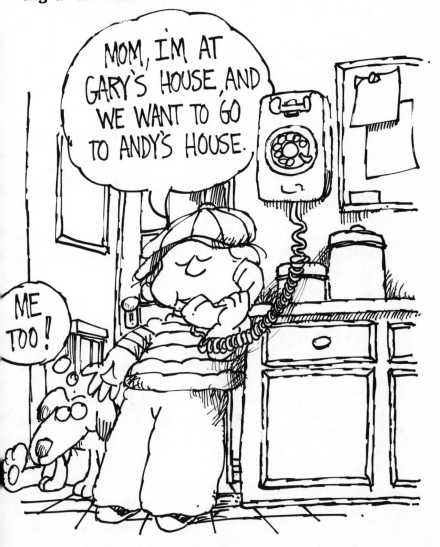

To make sure your parents or guardians know this:

1. Go straight to the place where you tell them you will be going to and stay there.

2. If you decide to go somewhere else on the way, call them and tell them where you are.

3. If you decide to go to another place after you have reached your destination, call your parents or guardians and tell them where you will be going.

4. If you are going to change your route in any way, let them know.

5. Be home when you say you will be home.

6. If you are going to be late, call your parents or guardians and let them know why you will be late and when you will be home.

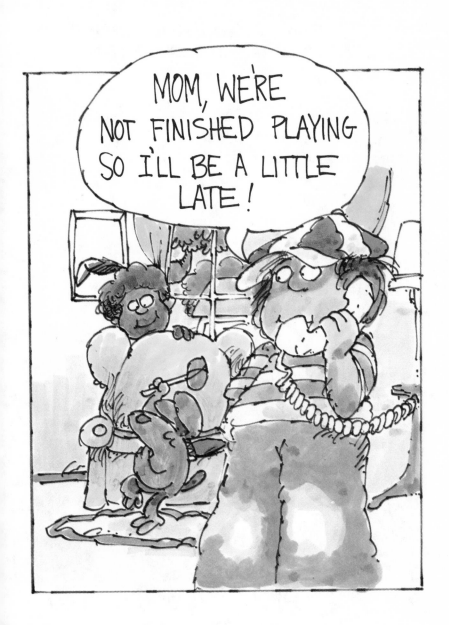

THINGS YOU NEED TO KNOW ABOUT YOUR PARENTS WHEN THEY ARE NOT HOME

You might find yourself facing an emergency in which you need your parents' help. If they are not home, you will need to know how you can reach them.

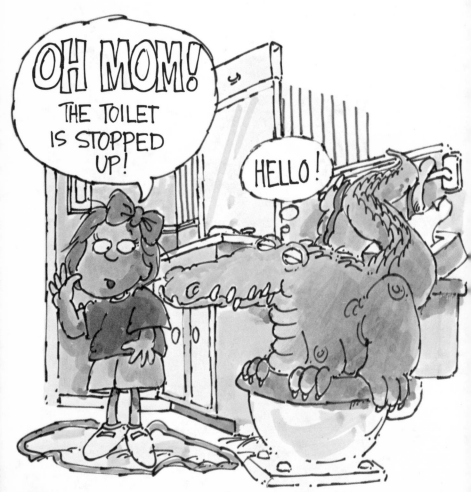

Before your parents leave, have them write down:

— where they are going (the name, address, and telephone number of the place),

— when they plan to return,

— whom to contact if they can't be reached (the name, address, and telephone number of the person).

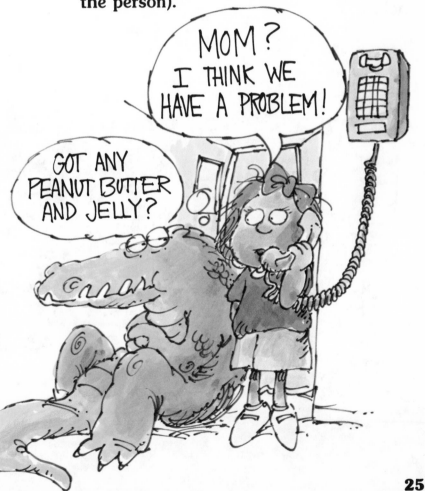

THINGS YOU NEED TO KNOW IN CASE OF EMERGENCIES IN WHICH YOU NEED SOMEONE BESIDES YOUR PARENTS OR GUARDIANS TO HELP YOU

You may face an emergency in which you will need someone besides your parents or guardians to help you. When this happens, you will need to know how to get in touch with the people who can help you.

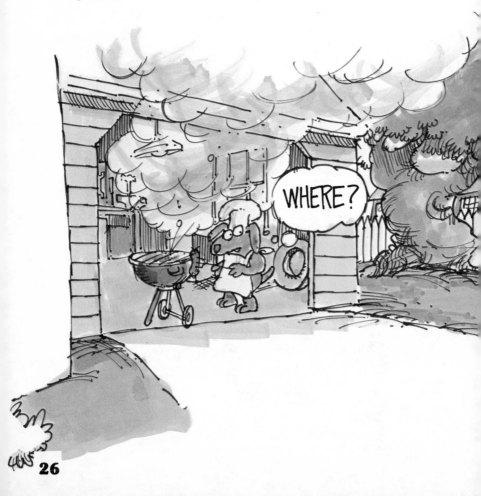

If someone is sick, you may need to call a doctor.

If someone is badly hurt, you may need to call a hospital, an ambulance, or the paramedics.

If someone has swallowed poison, you may need to call a poison control center.

If someone or something is threatening to harm you or your property, you may need to call the police.

If there is a fire, you may need to call the fire department.

If you need to get help, you will need to do it quickly. You will not want to spend time looking up phone numbers. To avoid this you should keep a list of emergency numbers near the phone. The list should be kept in plain sight at all times.

Here are some of the numbers your list should include:

dad (at work),
mom (at work),
friend or neighbor to contact if mom or dad
 can't be reached,
doctor,
dentist,
pharmacy,
emergency hospital,
ambulance,
paramedic,
poison control center,
police,
fire.

You may also want to include these numbers on the list:

taxi,   emergency shelter,
electric company,   gas company,
telephone company,   water company.

When you call someone to ask for help, it is important that you give them a message they can understand and remember.

This means you need to speak

    carefully,
    clearly, and
    accurately,

and don't hang up until they have all the information they need!

THIS IS BOBBY JONES. I'M CALLING ABOUT AN EMERGENCY INVOLVING A FIRE IN THE GARAGE AT 7236 LAUREL DRIVE, LOS ANGELES. THE TELEPHONE NUMBER IS (213) 555-4262. PLEASE COME AS SOON AS POSSIBLE!

It's a good idea to have an emergency sheet like this posted by your list of emergency telephone numbers so that you will be sure to give all of the correct information.

This is _____. I am calling about
　　　　　　　your name

an emergency involving a _____
　　　　　　　　　　　　　describe the emergency

_____

at _____
　　house address　　　　　　　　name of street

_____.
　　name of city

The nearest cross street is _____.

The telephone number here is _____
　　　　　　　　　　　　　　　　　　area code

_____.
phone number

Whenever you give this information, be sure that you do not waste time by giving a long description of the emergency. Keep your message short and to the point. Here are some examples of short descriptions.

I am calling about an emergency involving:

— a three-year-old child who is throwing up.

— a boy who fell off his bike and might have broken a leg.

— a baby who has eaten a whole bottle of aspirins.

— a person who is prowling in the backyard.

— a fire in the bedroom.

To make sure you can give the necessary information carefully, clearly, and accurately, practice with someone.

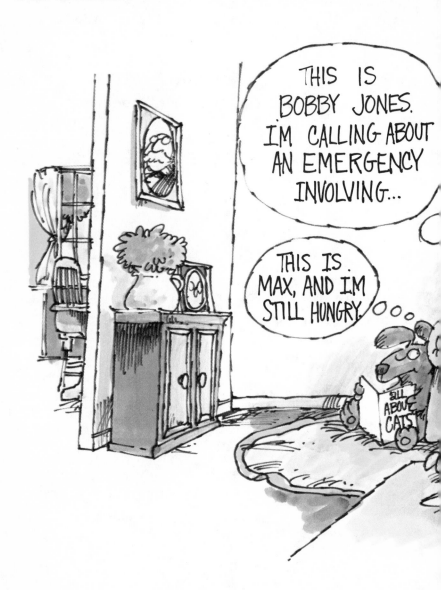

Pretend to call them. Give them the message and see if they can understand it.

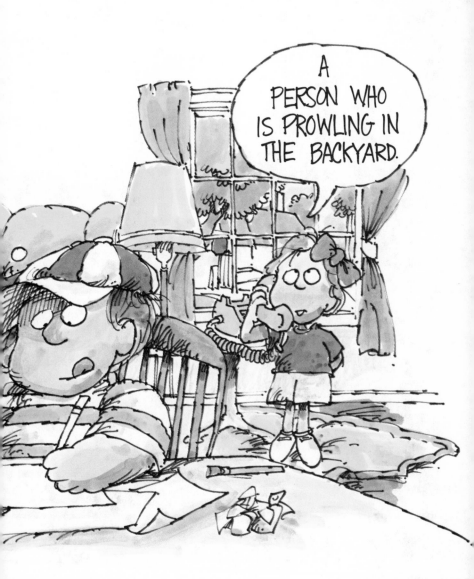

THINGS TO HAVE AT HOME

There are certain things every home **should have** so the people in it can deal with emergencies.

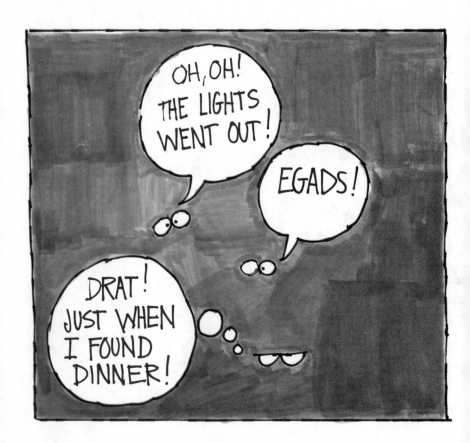

These things should be kept in places that everyone (except babies and very young children) can get to, and everyone should know exactly where they are.

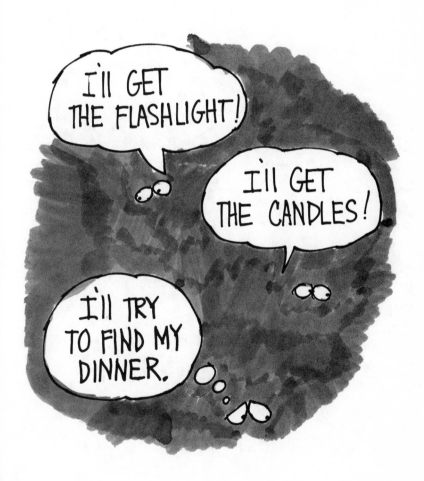

Every home should be provided with at least one flashlight.

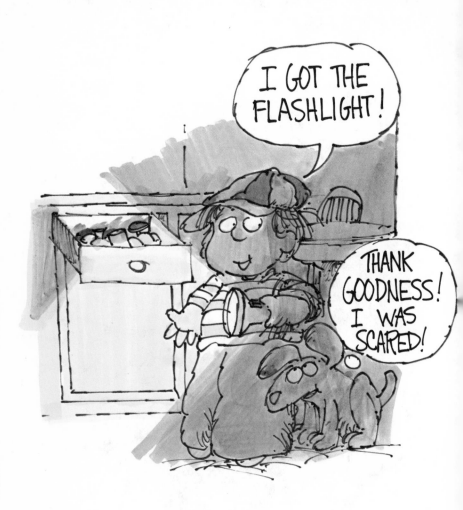

Another necessity every home needs is several candles and matches to light them with.

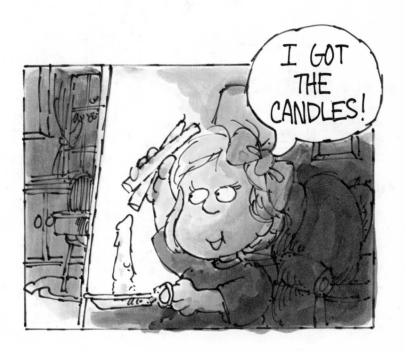

Every home should be equipped with a smoke alarm ...

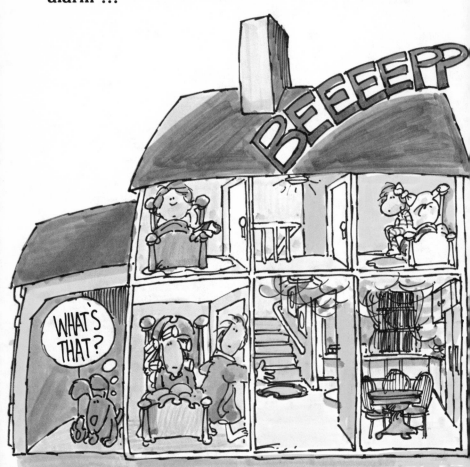

and a fire extinguisher and a garden hose that is always hooked up to a water faucet.

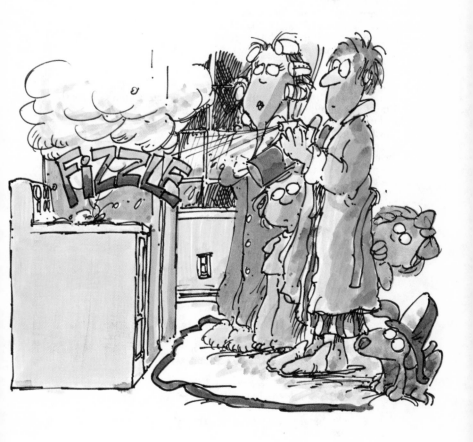

FIZZLE

Every home also needs medical supplies, including:

Activated charcoal (to absorb poison in case of poisoning)
Absorbent cotton
Adhesive strip bandage, assorted sizes
Adhesive tape, ½″ to 1″ wide
Ammonia inhalant (for fainting)
Antiseptic ointment
Anti-chapping ointment
Aspirin
Baking soda (for insect bites, poison oak, upset stomachs)
Boric acid solution (for cleaning wounds or rinsing out the eyes)
Butterfly bandages
Calamine lotion (for insect bites or poison oak)
Cotton-tipped swabs
Cough medicine (for coughs)
Drinking cups
Epsom salts (a strong laxative or used for soaking)
Eyedropper
Heating pad (to ease pain caused by sore muscles, cramps, etc.)
Hot water bottle (same use as a heating pad)
Hydrogen peroxide (to clean wounds)
Ice bag (to decrease swelling)
Insect bite lotion or repellent
Large triangular bandage
Laxative (for constipation)
Matches
Measuring cup
Measuring spoons
Oil of cloves (for toothaches)
Rubbing alcohol (to clean wounds and relieve high fevers)
Safety pins
Salt or salt tablets (for heat exhaustion)
Sharp sterilized needles (to remove splinters)
Sharp scissors with rounded edges
Soda mint tablets (for upset stomachs)
Special medication for individuals (prescribed by a doctor)
Sterile eye pads
Sterile gauze bandages - assorted sizes ½″ to 2″ wide
Sterile gauze pads 2″ × 4″
Syrup of Ipecac (to induce vomiting in case of poisoning)
Thermometer (rectal for infants)
Tongue depressors
Tourniquet with a short sturdy stick and a clean cloth 2″ wide and 2″ long
Tweezers

Children should not use medical supplies without the supervision of an adult! All medicines should be used only as directed by a doctor.

Your family may also need to have one or both of these special kits:

a snakebite kit to use if a person gets bitten by a poisonous snake ...

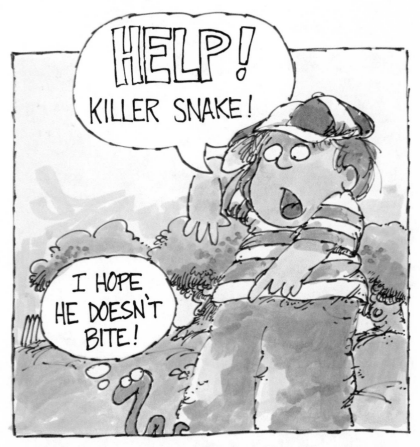

and an insect sting kit to be used by people who are very allergic to insect bites. You need a doctor's prescription to get this kit.

Every home should have a medical record for each person in the family. The medical record should include:

Person's name _____ Age _____

Birthdate _____

The doctor who cares
for this person _____ _____
                        Name   Address

_____
        Telephone number

Dates of the most recent immunizations:

Tetanus _____ Diphtheria _____

Polio _____ Measles _____

Blood Type _____ RH Factor _____

Other _____

Present medical problems and chronic conditions:

_____

Allergies (to drugs, insect bites, etc.):

_____

Medications taken regularly: _____

Special precautions and other information: _____

_____

You should be familiar with all of the information
on your medical record and a copy of the record
should be kept on file at your school and any
other place where you spend a great deal of time.

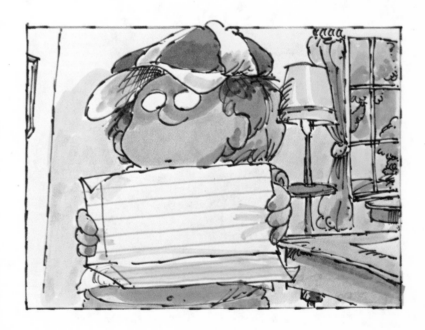

Every home should have a complete first aid book,

and everyone in the family should have a basic understanding of the information in the book.

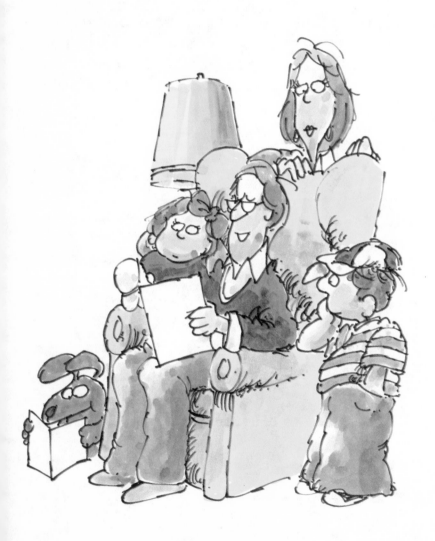

The car you travel in should carry a flashlight, emergency flares, and a small first aid kit.

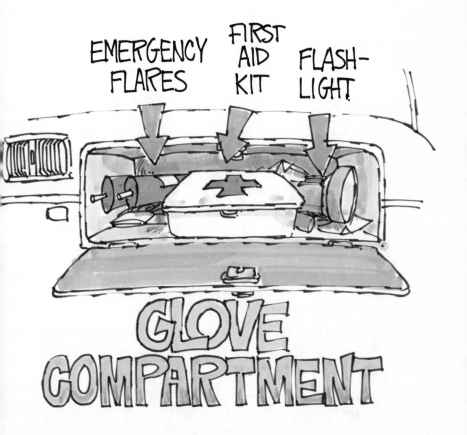

EMERGENCY FLARES

FIRST AID KIT

FLASH-LIGHT

GLOVE COMPARTMENT

THINGS TO HAVE AWAY FROM HOME

You should always try to carry identification, which includes your name, address, telephone number, blood type, and information about any special medical problems you have. You may want to carry an identification card in your pocket, purse, wallet, or knapsack, or you may want to wear your identification information around your neck, wrist, or ankle.

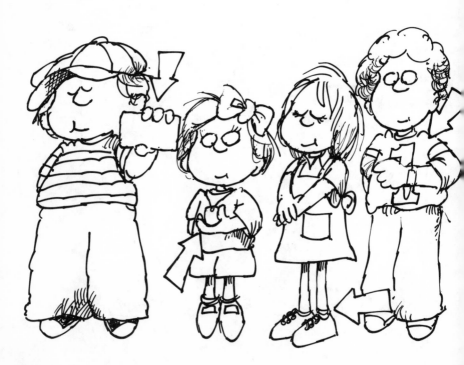

When you are away from home, you should always have enough money with you to make a telephone call home or to someone else who can help you.

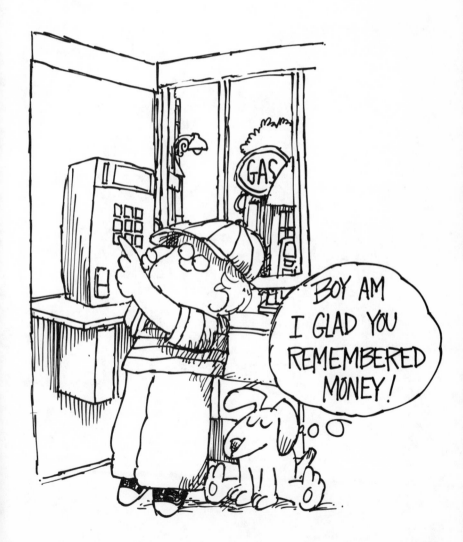

THE END of being unprepared.

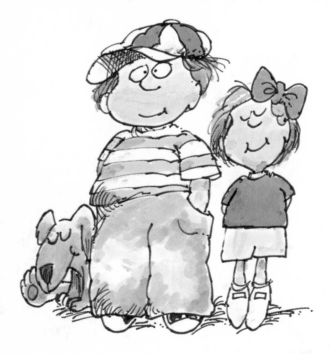